Natural sleep and its regulation

Dr Taylor Madison – Darwin E. – Richardson B. W.

Natural Sleep and its Regulation

LM Publishers

I – Sleep and its regulation[1]

Sleep as a factor in physical economics ranks in importance with respiration and digestion. Those who live normally, who throughout all ordinary exigencies maintain a natural attitude toward life, its strains and responsibilities, may expect to enjoy a full measure of this restorative function. How much each one needs is not to be determined by dogmatic rules or precedents, nor does each one require the same amount under every condition or circumstance. There must be enough, daily and weekly, and of suitable character, to restore the balance of neural energy reduced by whatsoever of fatigue follows upon daily activities; otherwise the sensorium resents this deprivation in one way or another. Individual needs vary and can only be determined inferentially, giving due weight to generally accepted requirements.

---

[1] By Dr Taylor Madison

Sleep, being the completest form of rest, is needed most by the youngest and least by the oldest. Most sleep is required by the weakest and least by the strongest. During childhood and exhaustive states too much sleep is rarely possible. For those in full tide of vigor too much sleep is often distinctly hurtful. Many modifications will immediately suggest themselves to those who are wise or learned in the science of bodily growth, development and disorders. Experience always counts for much. Variants, sometimes wide, are often permissible. Large errors will arise when these qualifications are marred by caprice, taste, prejudice; and harm follows, of one sort or another, sometimes of serious degree, by obscuration of sane reasoning on what may seem to be obvious and simple facts.

Physical efficiency depends chiefly upon the kind and amount of effort expended. Rest is an inevitable corollary. Relaxation is the starting point of all effort. For example, the strongest blows, the most accurate thrusts, can only proceed from an arm in thorough equipoise. Equipoise presupposes a full quantum of energy. Animal energy depends upon adequate rest as much as on force-giving foods. Complex acts, conditional always upon harmonies between intact central nervous dynamos, and well-adjusted mechanisms, can only be performed in their completeness when forces are at the norm.

Sleep is an absolute necessity for conscious beings. There are those who oppose this view, and some require relatively little, and that too, for long periods. Some sleep lightly, retaining in greater part their consciousness. Occasionally we hear of an individual who has lived for a long time without sleep, so far as can be determined, and yet has continued to maintain good health. Sufferers from one form or another of nervous exhaustion are often compelled to forego sleep temporarily. Vigorous persons of pronounced personality and highly developed consciousness have the least need for sleep, at least while at the zenith of their powers and in the full flower of energizing.

The maintenance of conscious life demands an expenditure of energy so intense that the processes of nutrition and reconstruction of cellular waste cannot be carried on without sleep. Complete repose of the consciousness is demanded for the plastic nutrition of the organism and the accomplishment of vegetative life. Consciousness is the highest of our faculties, rendering possible moral and scientific ideation; it demands the greatest efforts of our organism. In its absence sleep is less required.

All the internal organs are, during sleep, relatively less filled with blood because then the skin is in a state of hyperemia or gorged with blood. The sweat glands act more energetically at night whether we are asleep or awake, hence the danger of chills is then greater. All the organic activities continue, but are less vigorous at night, and during sleep, whereas during sleep in daylight hours these proceed with little alteration. When animals or men feel the desire to sleep they instinctively seek a quiet sheltered spot, as free as possible from light and noise, thus avoiding whatever impressions from the external world are liable to be subjectively translated into sensations. The eyelids are lowered; a position is sought wherein the muscles can be fully relaxed. The sensorial organs are capable of acting during sleep and continue to transmit impressions into conscious sensations.

With the pallor of the brain, which occurs in sleeping animals, the cortex ceases to react so readily to mechanical, photic, electric or other stimuli. The spinal cord and sensory nerves do not sleep, yet sensations of pain are then lowered. The nerves transmit painful impressions, but the consciousness of the sleeper perceives them incompletely. The voluntary muscles become quiescent during sleep, but retain their power, as shown by the normal subject in changing position, arranging the bedclothes, even walking; soldiers are able to march or ride while asleep. The brain is the chief part which sleeps, but it is not wholly inactive, exciting inhibitions which check the formation of reflex movements. If stimuli are applied of sufficient intensity to overcome the protective states of the somnolent consciousness the subject awakes, recognizing the cause more or less certainly.

Sleep is not an absolute arrest of cerebral activity; the brain then retains always partial energy. In deprivation of sleep it is the brain which suffers most, while in deprivation of food it is the brain which preserves longest the integrity of its structure and function. In young animals, abundantly fed and cared for but kept awake, there follows serious lesions of the organism which soon become irreparable, and death results.

There have been many theories and hypotheses advanced to explain the phenomena of somnolence. The physiologists have here, as so frequently elsewhere, exhibited far more academic than practical interest in the matter. There is no subject, however, of greater importance, since it is a prime factor in all the reparative phenomena of life, standing at the foundation of nutrition; yet no research work has been done on the nature of sleep commensurate with the gravity of the subject. Psychologists have written extensively on one phenomenon of sleep, viz., dreams. Normal sleep has attracted so little attention that we do not know exactly how to modify it in accordance with common conditions of bodily derangements. Inferentially certain facts seem established which not only account for the phenomena of sleep, but enable us to reason from them and thus to regulate the state in great measure; sometimes sufficiently. It is probable that during sleep there is a diminished resistance in the surface vessels, inducing lowered blood pressure, hence smaller amounts of blood pass through the brain. As sleep approaches the cerebral vessels grow relatively less filled with blood for an hour or more after full somnolence has come. After reaching its minimum tension the brain circulation remains practically constant for one or two hours or more, gradually returning to normal as the time for awakening nears.

After having attained a fair idea of what sleep is, whereby we can better appreciate a reasoning from our individual standpoint, we may proceed to discuss its regulation. For the young, who may be assumed to be in possession of full neural and circulatory balance, whether in or out of health, the regulation of sleep is a simple matter, one which will in most instances adjust itself if the subject be placed under normal conditions.

We may fix our attention most profitably upon the status of sleep in those of middle or late life. Here a number of causes conspire to disturb equilibrium of body cells, sometimes slightly, and at others it will be found that effects have been insidiously wrought which may suddenly obtrude upon our attention, causing great distress, often impairing the integrity of our judgment, hence our working efficiency. Therefore a double peril assails. Mere inability to sleep naturally, or as heretofore, or as each one assumes as a right, is, especially among men (who shrink from admission of physical weakness), seldom regarded as worth their seeking the advice of a physician. Whereupon the simplest remedy is to hunt about for something which will obtund the consciousness. Often this is a form of alcohol. A friend will advise a glass of whiskey at bedtime, may be two or more; beer is popular for this purpose; some special form of wine is often recommended, and (deplorable as it may seem) too often by the physician.

The entering wedge is so easy, and in the main agreeable in its primary effects, that the habit of tippling is thus readily established. Or again the chemists' shops are filled with ' simple harmless remedies for insomnia.' The sign boards in all public places glisten with advice. Every acquaintance is ready with counsel, especially those numerous well intentioned women with little else to do but to prattle of their shallow convictions on matters coming within the narrow range of their experience, medical, spiritual or social. It is never safe to play with drugs; to trifle with agencies often hurtful to a pro- found degree in their ultimate effects. Idiosyncracies exist, too, whereby what may harm one not at all produces in another far-reaching derangements of vital organs. One of the most dangerous lunatics I ever saw was a man possessed by sudden homicidal tendencies. He would have remained so had not it been discovered, by providential accident, that he was accustomed to use habitually moderately large doses of some bromide. The obsession promptly and permanently disappeared by total withdrawal and the use of an antidote. We physicians, especially those who see many instances of nervous derangements, are constantly coming in contact with the deplorable derangements caused by hypnotic drugs, many of which are ordinarily classed as innocent. The action of narcotics presents none of the characteristics of normal sleep except the temporary arrest of consciousness; hence narcosis is not true sleep. It does not refresh and regenerate vigor as does normal sleep. To be sure, drug unconsciousness may and often does pass into sleep. Again there are those who have be- come so accustomed to narcotics that, when deprived of them, they cannot sleep. This would seem to prove a sort of antagonism between the drug effect and natural sleep. In brief, whatever agents inhibit cerebral activity, inducing local anemia, hence permitting sleep or narcosis, are harmless provided they do not derange nutrition or cause other ill effects. All narcotic drugs invite these evil effects in varying degrees and hence are to be avoided, and only used in extreme cases and under guidance of a competent physician.

The other peril lies in the fact that derangements of sleep often foreshadow serious structural damage of the heart, arteries or other organs or tissues. Hence unless the phenomena be estimated intelligently, in the light of other than obvious data only to be secured through careful medical examination, a deadly disease process may escape detection until too late to accomplish full repair.

To secure regular consecutive sleep it is best to assume that position which is most natural and best suited to invite the least disturbance of the functions of the great organs. To use the analogy of the four-footed animals, and by such facts we can secure the safest guidance, the best position is on the abdomen or nearly so. Habits may, and do, vitiate our instincts here as elsewhere, and we can accustom ourselves to many departures from natural and advisable operations. This is especially forceful while in vigorous health, but we are speaking here of securing the best rest with the least tax upon our organism, hence it is well to determine those means which are normal, and employ them. The body should lie as nearly as possible on a level, head and feet as well as body, on the side inclined toward the abdomen, adjusting arms and legs in such a fashion as shall not permit undue pressure upon nerves and bloodvessels, direct or indirect.

To lie on the back is objectionable for the reason that long continued pressure on the tissues adjacent to the vertebral column, which are innervated by the posterior primary divisions of the spinal nerves, exerts a continued irritation through vasomotor connections to the viscera, disturbing the circulation in the segments. Here are the cell bodies of the vasomotor nerves, which thence pass to the organs and beyond parts, thereby governing function. Thus, dilatation is induced and maintained in the blood vessels of the viscera. Also certain results follow directly by effect of gravity. Pressure on the abdominal organs, and their varying contents, is exerted upon the great vessels, arterial, venous and lymphatic, the sympathetic plexuses, and the ebb and flow of fluid in them is deranged. Hence function and nutrition of these structures are influenced unfavorably. Man is the only animal which sleeps on the back. This attitude should only be assumed for short periods. During extreme weakness this position is often taken, but it is the duty of attendants to urge a frequent change to the side, otherwise several hurtful effects may follow, among which the least grave are nightmare and evil dreams. The poisons of katabolism circulating in the blood tend to be deposited in the outlying tissues ; hence arise pneumonia and bedsores. Not only is this true for those who are suffering from one or another form of disability, but for those in robust health, especially when sleeping on the back after full meals. Many obscure forms of digestive or circulatory disorders may have been initiated in infancy through lying too long upon the back.

In animals, among whom such disorders are rare and whose spinal column is constantly horizontal, there is little or no change in the relative positions of the great organs at any time. In man, who is constantly altering the relationships of these viscera by lying, standing, stooping, the blood supply and venous return are subject to frequent interruptions, and strains are exerted upon the supporting structures of the blood vessels and thus the vasomotor mechanisms are taxed heavily. The head should be permitted to rest as nearly upon a level as the feet, though most people prefer some support. The blood should be encouraged to reach all parts of the body equally, hence the limbs had best be extended, not flexed ; the habit of extending the arms above the head is a particularly bad one.

To secure the most perfect repose the temperature of all parts should be equalized before retiring. Cold feet induce delay in securing sleep and it is then shallow when attained. The bladder and bowels by weight of their contents will interfere with repose, hence they should be previously emptied. It is most unwise to overfill the stomach before retiring; this disturbs sleep almost as much as hunger, but moderate eating before sleeping is not hurtful, and is often salutary.

Sleep is only a function; therefore, whatever disturbs it depends on structural derangement of some sort. Disorders of sleep are manifold. The commonest are psychic exaltations or depressions, worries, brooding on the cares of the day, continuing to dwell on the waking problems. Habit is ever forceful. A well-trained mind will promptly shut off or readily let go of the thought processes. Unnatural activity of the sensory and association centers causes dreams ; that of the motor centers results in shocks, starts and spasmodic phenomena. Control of the visceral centers may become inhibited, permitting unconscious discharges from the bladder, intestines or sexual organs; innervation of the lungs or heart being thus deranged, palpitation or dyspnoea is induced. Sensory centers being over-stimulated, sensations of light follow, or of sound, also pain or vertigo. " In fine, the ordinary smooth current of the subconscious activities breaks against some pathologic states and now one symptom, now another, is thrust out and so unpleasantly that the sleeper awakens" (C. L. Dana).

A review of Dana's remarks on the disorders of sleep will be useful to achieve an understanding of the varieties and phenomena of insomnia; a better term perhaps would be difficulties of sleep. Some people, especially those of middle age, fall asleep easily, but wake in the small hours and thereafter only doze fitfully. This may be due to beginning degenerative changes in the arteries, connected with the effects of worries and strains, or only a habit, or echo of youthful customs of early rising, or an acquired weakness or irritability of the heart. Others fall asleep readily, but are soon disturbed by little explosions of motor, sensory or psychic forces. The body or limbs start or jerk; sleep follows, but these nervous explosions may be repeated two or three times. It is usually the result of exhaustion, psychic or muscular over-tension, physiologic irritability, indigestion, nervous fatigue, or may foreshadow some serious derangement. Sudden awakenings often betray emotional distress, fear or disorders of ideation.

Weir Mitchell has written fascinatingly of disorders of sleep, making absorbing reading for the profession as well as the laity. He it was who described first the sensory shocks, strange feelings passing along the body, culminating in some abrupt explosion, noise, odor or vision. Vertigo is occasionally thus experienced, especially by those who have felt it before. That mysterious malady called ' migraine' sometimes occurs suddenly while asleep ' and hales the sufferer from profound sleep to waking hours of misery.'

Morbid or perverted sensations, numbness, ' pins and needles ' fornications and such like mild neuroses appear at times during sleep. Limbs may seem ' dead,' sensation being temporarily lost and not in any way which follows upon marked pressure interrupting the flow of nervous impulses, but purely a phenomenon of sleep. These are more common in the later hours of night, when the motor cells are restored in part, losing irritability, the sensory cells being still excitable. These discomforts may be referred to interruptions in the conductivity of the spinal cord. Nocturnal psychoses, the night terrors of children, nightmare, strange mental vagaries, changes in intellectual and emotional balance, are of such wide variety that they can only be alluded to ; each person of rich experience is able to recall instances. In these conditions of distress much folly can be committed, and frequently is; evil thoughts are thus engendered, which too often influence action later. Sometimes imperative impulses arising in slumber drive one to commit questionable or silly deeds. The imagination in some is thus stimulated to utter weird statements, or to put on record what are falsely estimated to be thoughts of deep significance. I recall reading an incident in the early official life of Bismarck, who often thus wakened in the night with the conviction that he had solved perplexing problems. On reducing to writing the ideas thus excited he found, on perusal next day, that they were altogether fanciful. It is true, valuable ideas do come in dreams or in real temporary waking states.

The sleep of early life is peculiarly sensitive to irritations of the organs below the diaphragm, digestive or genital ; in later life to those above, of the heart, blood vessels or lungs. In this connection we may refer to dreams. The suspension of brain activity in sleep is only partial; there prevails a certain amount of psychic life. Every nervous stimulus, sensation or idea leaves an impression, a trace, in the cerebrospinal system. Obscure motions, influences, irritants generated in the organism, may afterward revive temporarily under some impulsation of consciousness, as by afflux of blood. Each cell of the body is endowed with more or less memory (Henle), for by this means are preserved hereditary influences, the transmission of psychic and mental characteristics, the after images of sensations. In this manner many sounds, sights, feelings, which are partially conveyed to the sensorium, may become revived and variously interpreted to the consciousness. Predormitial sensations, thoughts and movements are thus capable of inducing multiplication and diverse auto-interpretation. Dreams grow luxuriantly when the state is one of partial wakefulness. The influences of the day are then woven into fanciful pictures more or less reflecting actual life.

If sleep be profound the imagination is no longer dominated by actualities and there arises the phenomenon of a special world, that of dreams. Mental activity is really physical activity; hence we may experience consequential fatigue. At the bottom of the emotion may be found a subjective excitation of the peripheral nervous apparatus. This form of reflected life constitutes the basis of dreaming, the imagination, hallucinations, the realm of fancy. Dreams have their origin in those parts of the organism most active in the waking state, in eyes, ears, the tactile, temperature and muscular sense. The same obtains as to hallucinations in the insane. A very deep sleep does not permit of dreams, or the waking memory cannot recall them, whereas in very light sleep dreams are frequent and can be remembered.

Dreams are more numerous and picturesque among intellectual people, and during certain exhaustive states, and less among those of lower mentality. The more primitive, young and intellectual the person, the more illogical, disjointed and elementary are the dreams. In old age, and profound depressive states, dreams are most rare; they serve many useful purposes. To the physician certain features of dreams possess a valuable significance. They exercise a salutary influence upon otherwise unused areas of the brain and permit the excursions, or, may be, formation, of the faculty of imagination (Manaciene). They act as a defense against the monotonies and trivialties of real life, for without them we should grow old much more rapidly (Novalis). Many writers, poets, scientists, philosophers, musicians, etc., testify to the value of dreams in piecing out their concepts, idealizations, weaving a woof of imagination invaluable to the completed thought.

It will be seen that the regulation of impaired sleep reaches back to causes most varied. Some are slight and superficial; others are due to deep-seated derangements or lesions, beginning or established. In practice, however, certain plain simple procedures usually suffice to bring about happy results. Beyond what these can accomplish, skilled medical aid should be sought and a careful search made for definite disorders, and systematic measures instituted to remove them consonant with the difficulties encountered. It is well to remember that the causes of wakefulness may be highly complex; slight factors often acting with equal forcefulness with those which theoretically should be greatest.

We are concerned in our efforts to regulate the resting period of the consciousness, with possible morbidity in two directions; too much or too little. Ordinarily it is assumed that the more one gets of sleep the better. This view is so generally accepted that the custom of some physicians, especially those who see much of illness in the extreme periods of life, to order food or employ active measures at regular hours, involving the waking of the patient, verges upon the danger line. Judgment must be exercised, and is well within the capabilities of a good nurse. Serious exhaustion has often followed needless interruptions of repose during exhaustive states.

It is entirely demonstrable that a variety of disorders may result from, or are indicated by, excessive somnolence, partly of developmental and partly of degenerative origin. During infancy sleeping must predominate over waking states, the unconscious reflex life over the conscious intellectual life. It should be remembered, however, that consciousness requires exercise for development. Monotonous measures, such as rocking, swinging, unmusical lullabies, may serve a salutary purpose occasionally, but can readily be carried too far, to the point of lowering normal temperature, inducing excessive anemia of the brain and disturbances of circulation. Sleep should come by opportunity, comfortable position and customary environment. Habits should be formed sufficient in themselves to invite repose. It ought not to be interrupted needlessly, nor forced by measures or drugs which obtund the consciousness. Normality of sleeping capacity is the product of intellectual equipoise. Stupid folk are proverbially dull, lethargic, with large capacities for deep sleep. Some part of this is no doubt the result of over indulgence. The consciousness is often enfeebled by disuse in young or old. In the young the impetus to exercise the faculties demands encouragement; also, as age enfeebles the brain structures, mental stagnation, hence degeneration, is invited by over- much time spent in unconsciousness. Nutritive balance, the expenditure of energy, cannot be maintained indefinitely. Renewals must occur, and it is shown that inordinate somnolence makes for exhaustion of body and mind; the kidneys suffer, their vessels become distended and hence enfeebled. In the aged the tone of the tissues, especially of the vessel walls, tends to become devitalized, leading to a stasis in lymph and blood vessels and to various forms of organic derangement. In deep sleep, long continued, this stasis of blood and lymph is unduly encouraged, sometimes to the point of paralysis. The bile becomes thickened, stagnated; the bowels, the intestines, suffer from a surfeit of sleep, impairing the machinery of peristalsis, hence follows constipation. The urinary organs also share in this derangement of elimination and gravel, calculi, may form. Anemias are often unaccountable, but it will be found that chlorotics usually sleep too much and are the better for its regulation.

There is no simple fact more forcefully borne in upon the writer than that early rising and movement in the open air before breakfast is a measure of vast importance in a large array of chronic ailments, especially those involving gout, dyspepsia, constipation, obesity and disorders of the sense organs. Many people aver that they are made miserable by rising early, stirring about before taking food, and consequently suffer from headaches, nausea, prostration and the like. These phenomena are the results of some derangements in the circulatory balance, most probably due to a morbid quality of sleep, which for the most part is remediable. In proof of this statement is the fact, usually clearly demonstrable, that if the physician can secure fair cooperation, with persistence all this wretchedness will disappear. Particularly is this shown if circumstances compel the patient to alter his habits for the better. Abundant illustrative instances could be cited. Weir Mitchell in his recommendations for the rest treatment, so valuable in the repair of profound conditions of exhaustion, compels a fixed hour for wakening, usually seven a.m. Often it has been the writer's duty to soothe and explain to Dr. Mitchell's patients, who resented being awakened, the reason for this regulation.

Disuse of muscle is followed by atrophy; so of other tissues. Strength can only grow by judicious, continued use. Witness the pitiable spectacle of steady degeneration in the tissues, in mental and physical aptitudes, commonly displayed in those of advancing years, who, through withdrawal of normal stimuli to exertion, permit their organs and their structures to fall into disuse. Prosperity, interpreted so often to mean cessation of energies, is often fatal to physical and mental efficiency. The antidote is simple and most effective, the retention of habits of usefulness applied all along the whole line of normal activities.

The whole range of bodily derangements and diseases can be interpreted through variations in the blood supply. This again depends upon the incidence of diverse irritants, infections from without or poisons generated within ; or such as are the products of changes in the blood plasma effecting oxygenation.

Sleep being the relaxation, suspension, of the consciousness, the brain being the center of consciousness, it naturally follows that, as evidence shows, the circulation in the brain is, during sleep, at the lowest normal tension. Whatever disturbs sleep, therefore, probably induces an afflux of blood to the brain. It is evident that to sleep peacefully and continually it is important that the blood pressure shall be as nearly as possible normal. If this be markedly above or below par sleep is interfered with. Plethoric folk, however, supposedly of over-tense vessels, often sleep better than the feeble and weakly; yet they are more likely to slumber heavily, are difficult to wake, and on waking suffer from morning confusion and headache; in short, are far less refreshed by their slumber and require longer to acquire waking balance than frail beings whose sleep is shallow, interrupted and seemingly insufficient.

All these facts and reasonings from vascular tone constitute a long, somewhat technical, story ; suffice it to say that, in order to secure comfortable natural sleep there is demanded a careful regulation of blood supply and distribution. Where a careful regulation of life fails to accomplish this, help must be sought of a wise physician, who will promptly determine what is amiss. The difficulty may be found to be due to faulty skin action, cold extremities, intestinal accumulations, or visceral poisons, organic derangements, a weak heart, an overtired body, an overwrought brain or other physical disorders, the province of the physician. Interference with matters out of the realm of our experience is usually followed by punishment. Among the most dangerous things a person can do is to take a shot in the dark and medical procedures, swallowing medicines on blind guesses. Damage must almost inevitably result, first by deranging digestion, perhaps already at fault, and next achieving stupor, not true sleep, or encouraging the brain to demand meretricious, unsuitable soporifics.

While it is most desirable that sleep should be taken in regular amounts, at a suitable time, and this during the hours of darkness and continuously, still it is possible that various habits may be formed, seemingly peculiar, which suffice for ordinary requirements. These may be acquired to meet some temporary demand, or become habitual for years. For instance, mothers of young babies commonly form the habit of sleeping and waking readily and frequently, and yet continue to enjoy excellent health. Trained nurses acquire even more complex, yet systematic, habits of sleep and wakefulness; a regular irregularity, yet productive of little or no exhaustion, at least for a time. Persons engaged in diverse strenuous occupations secure a power of seizing sleep when they can get it, notably sailor men by ' watches ' of four hours each, twice a day.

Sleep, being the chief restorative agency for the consciousness, the desideratum is chiefly to achieve enough repose in sufficient completeness to effect repair of brain cells and other centers of energy. In those whose lives are full of repeated and emphatic demands upon them for concentration of attention, the habit of taking short naps is found to be most refreshing and invigorating. Many physicians, some lawyers, and other professional men who pursue literary work, find it satisfactory to secure a brief sleep some time during the day, often in the middle of operations, when an opportunity offers. Thus a short sleep in a chair, or preferably lying down on the back on a bench or lounge, will rejuvenate the powers and permit intellectual work far into the night. While a certain number of hours of consecutive sleep are imperative for full health, these cannot be dogmatically determined except by carefully weighing circumstances, which vary. Lumber men on the ' drive ' maintain excellent health on the smallest amount of sleep, during the most trying circumstances, after intense physical exertion so long as the spring daylight lasts, often wet to the skin, with little or no bedclothes or protection at night from freezing weather and fed irregularly, often insufficiently. Armies, exploring parties and others have similar experiences, and suffer no distress for days and weeks, the men often actually gaining in health, seldom losing. If the circumstances be cheerful, such competition, overcoming the forces of nature, is salutary. If peril, strained attention or tyrannous officers complicate the conditions, ill health may appear early and is then often severe.

When to sleep is again a matter of opinion. Early rising is by common consent a salutary custom, especially when the day comes early, not otherwise. It is agreed that more sleep is required in winter than in summer. The best sleep is had during the hours of darkness. The mind is clearest in the early morning, and those who can utilize this period for intellectual work are capable of turning out the best products. Some cannot do so, or think they cannot, and yet furnish excellent results.

The sleeping room should be cool, abundant air being always ad- mitted. This should not be interpreted to mean that the room may safely remain intensely cold. In the modern treatment of tuberculosis fresh air is recognized to be imperatively needed all day and all night. Artificial heat can, and should, be supplied along with the fresh air, till the temperature of the room be at or near 50° F. or 55° F., for some even 60° F. Above this no one in health is likely to sleep in perfect comfort. Babies and invalids need a heat of from 60° F. to 70° F., even more at times, yet all require the fresh air, or fullest ventilation.

Fever patients, even those suffering from pneumonia or bronchitis, may sleep with safety and great advantage in a thoroughly ventilated cool room and with no more covering on them than is needed for protection from sudden changes of temperature which might send their body heat down below normal. It is needless to particularize as to the offensiveness, deleteriousness, of the body and lung exhalations emitted by those asleep. This is more than apparent, it is actually greater by far than when awake, and demands prompt removal and an abundance of good air to replace that which is vitiated. There are those who still cling to the shred of demon influence which causes them to ' dread the night air ' when spirits range and goblins weave evil spells; when diseases come wafting in at open windows, keyholes and other joints in the harness of defense. Since the pestiferous mosquito has been proved the chief carrier of mephitic paludal diseases, insect nettings are deemed sufficient to ward off evil nocturnal influences. Sleeping in a close exhausted atmosphere is so promptly and painfully punished by discomforts, that it would seem there could not be two minds on the matter. Yet many refined and educated folk still prefer the shut windows. Curiously enough some woods-men, farmers and others who live much in the open air incline to a hot room for sleeping. To my sorrow, I have often been compelled to experience this prejudice.

Body clothing at night should be loose, not dense, permitting the ready passage of air, never of wool next to the skin. Bed clothing should not be too close of texture, blankets being preferable to dense ' comfortables ' and not ' tucked in ' too closely. Air should be allowed to pass occasionally under the sides at least as one turns about more or less freely. I have proved this in open camps in bitter temperatures, thus using less clothing than those who slept in bags. Indian guides often sleep with their heads covered and their feet bare to the fire. Even on the long trail I prefer pajamas to close fitting day underwear at night. Under these circumstances, too, occasionally rising and warming by a fire gives better rest than to stay close in a sleeping bag all night long. As to beds the firm mattress with springs is vastly better than soft clinging surfaces.

Some people sleep with a profundity, a completeness, from which they can only be aroused with difficulty. They occasionally wake unrefreshed with confusion, headaches, stiffness and soreness of limbs. This is unfortunate and usually betokens some abnormality in health which should be corrected. Such deep somnolence is not so restorative as the lighter forms of slumber. Again limbs become cramped, hence nerves and blood vessels suffer hurtful pressure, by long remaining in one position; the integrity of the internal organs likewise is imperiled. Sleep is invited by darkness. Light, even though the eyes be closed, penetrates the lids and stirs the consciousness through these most delicate of sense organs. Hence it is wise to exclude light if one must sleep after the sun has risen. A useful device is to cover the eyes with black cloth or even a handkerchief folded, or use a screen, rather than to exclude daylight from the entire room, which too often means exclusion of air as well. Those whose heart and arteries lack tone may give attention to this to secure or to maintain sleep. Day drowsiness and night wakefulness indicate often a cardiac weakness demanding attention. Conversely, high pulse is usually present in those who sleep over heavily.

A complete circulatory balance is needed for those who would sleep most refreshingly. One of the best means to secure this is by exercise at bedtime, enough to distribute the blood to the surface and muscles, hence to relieve the tension in the vessels of the brain. High vascular tension is often a cause of insomnia ; it may be continuous or only due to psychic causes, worries, morbid tension, over-excited circulation or toxins. Hence the common device of the hot foot bath, hot entire bath, or even a cold bath inducing reaction, may suffice. To execute some systematic movements with little or no clothing on is better; in cold weather with extra clothing on, such as a sweater. Certain movements, especially those of the neck and shoulders, are particularly useful. A series of movements I devised in treating a chronic neurosis put many patients promptly to sleep. Also certain manipulations of the neck, especially a distributed pressure over the posterior occipital nerves, have in certain cases of obstinate insomnia in my hands been followed by complete cure. One man who claimed he had not slept a full night for thirty years was thus put to sleep in my office and after a course of treatment he remained free from this distress. That admirable instrument, now unfortunately out of fashion, the bicycle, cured scores of insomniacs by affording patients the means of prompt lowering of blood pressure by a ride just before bedtime. Few measures are more prompt, certain and permanent.

Eating some light food is often of value, but the overfull stomach is frequently a cause of shallow or distressed sleep. There are many forms of digestive derangement, liver troubles, toxemias, etc., which impair sleep in those who are under the impression they have powerful digestions. Nothing wakes some people so certainly at evil hours as an over-acid stomach, relievable by a simple alkali or charcoal. The bowels are best evacuated before bedtime; if full they may cause much loss of sleep. In short, as Emerson says of all health, of which sleep is a major item, it is not to be bought, it must be earned; and wisdom, frugality, self restraint, industry, perhaps all cardinal virtues, con- tribute to this boon.

II – The Physiology of sleep[2]

Perfect sleep is the possession, as a rule, of childhood only. The healthy child, worn out with its day of active life, suddenly sinks to rest, sleeps its ten or twelve hours, and wakes, believing, feeling, that it has merely closed its eyes and opened them again; so deep is its twinkle of oblivion. The sleep in this case is the nearest of approaches to actual death, and at the same time presents a natural paradox, for it is the evidence of strongest life.

During this condition of perfect sleep, what are the physiological conditions of the sleeper? Firstly, all the senses are shut up, yet are they so lightly sealed that the communication of motion by sound, by mechanical vibration, by communication of painful impression, is sufficient to unseal the senses, to arouse the body, to renew all the proofs of existing active life. Secondly, during this period of natural sleep the most important changes of nutrition

---

[2] by Richardson B. W.

are in progress; the body is renovating, and, if young, is actually growing; if the body be properly covered, the animal heat is being conserved and laid up for expenditure during the waking hours that are to follow; the respiration is reduced, the inspirations being lessened in the proportion of six to seven as compared with the number made when the body is awake; the action of the heart is reduced; the voluntary muscles, relieved of all fatigue and with the extensors more relaxed than the flexors, are undergoing repair of structure and recruiting their excitability; and the voluntary nervous system, dead for the time to the external vibration, or as the older men called it "stimulus" from without, is also undergoing rest and repair, so that when it comes again into work it may receive better the impressions it may have to gather up, and influence more effectively the muscles it may be called upon to animate, direct, control.

Thirdly, although in the organism during sleep there is suspension of muscular and nervous power, there is not universal suspension; a narrow, but at the same time safe, line of distinction separates the sleep of life from the sleep of death. The heart is a muscle, but it does not sleep, and the lungs are worked by muscles, and these do not sleep; and the viscera which triturate and digest food are moved by muscles, and these do not sleep; and the glands have an arrangement for the constant separation of fluids, and the glands do not sleep; and all these parts have certain nerves which do not sleep. These all rest, but they do not cease their functions. Why is it so?

The reason is that the body is divided into two systems as regards motion. For every act of the body we have a system of organs under the influence of the will, the voluntary, and another system independent of the will, the involuntary. The muscles which propel the body, and are concerned in all acts we essay to perform, are voluntary; the muscles, such as the heart and the stomach, which we cannot control, are involuntary. Added to these are muscles which, though commonly acting involuntarily, are capable of being moved by the will: the muscles which move the lungs are of this order, for we can if we wish suspend their action for a short time or quicken it; these muscles we call semi-voluntary. In sleep, then, the voluntary muscles sleep, and the nervous organs which stimulate the voluntary muscles sleep; but the involuntary and the semi-voluntary muscles and their nerves merely rest: they do not veritably sleep.

This arrangement will be seen, at once, to be a necessity, for upon the involuntary acts the body relies for the continuance of life. In disease the voluntary muscles may be paralyzed, the brain may be paralyzed, but, if the involuntary organs retain their power, the animal is not dead. Sir Astley Cooper had under his care a man who had received an injury of the skull causing compression of the brain, and the man lay for weeks in a state of persistent unconsciousness and repose; practically he slept. He did not die, because the involuntary system remained true to its duty; and, when the great surgeon removed the compression from the brain of the man, the sleeper woke from his long trance and recovered. Dr. Wilson Philip had a young dog that had no brain, and the animal lay in profound insensibility for months, practically asleep; but the involuntary parts continued uninfluenced, and the animal lived and, under mechanical feeding, grew fat. Flourens had a brainless fowl that lived in the same condition. It neither saw nor heard, he says, nor smelled nor tasted nor felt; it lost even its instincts; for however long it was left to fast, it never voluntarily ate; it never shrunk when it was touched, and, when attacked by its fellows, it made no attempt at self-defense, neither resisting nor escaping. In fine, it lost every trace of intelligence, for it neither willed, remembered, felt, nor judged: yet it swallowed food when the food was put into its mouth, and fattened. In these cases, as in that of the injured man, the involuntary systems sustained the animal life. It is the same in sleep.

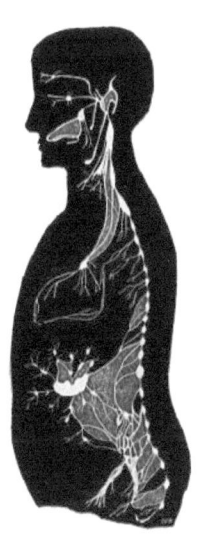

When we look at these phenomena, as anatomists, we find a reason for them in structure and character of parts. The involuntary muscles have a special anatomical structure; and the nervous organism that keeps the involuntary muscles in action is a distinct organism. There are, briefly, two nervous systems: one locked up in the bony cavity of the skull and in the bony canal of the spine, with nerves issuing there from to the muscles; and another lying within the cavities of the body, with nerves issuing from it to supply all the involuntary muscles. The first of these systems, consisting of the brain, the spinal cord, and the nerves of sense, sensation, and motion, is called the cerebro-spinal or voluntary system of nerves; the second, consisting of a series of nervous ganglia with nerves which communicate with the involuntary muscles and with nerves of the voluntary kind, is called, after Harvey the vegetative, after Bichat the organic system: a sketch of this organic system is depicted in the accompanying diagram.

In sleep, the cerebro-spinal system sleeps; the organic system retains its activity. Thus in sleep the voluntary muscles and parts fail to receive their nervous stimulation; but the involuntary receive theirs still, and under it move in steady motion; while the semi-voluntary organs also receive sufficient stimulation to keep them in motion.

Of all the involuntary organs, the heart, which is the citadel of motion, is most protected. To itself belongs a special nervous centre, that which feeds it steadily with stimulus for motion; from the cervical ganglia of the organic nervous system it receives a second or supplementary supply; and from the brain it receives a third supply, which, passive under ordinary circumstances, can under extraordinary circumstances become active and exert a certain controlling power. Then the arteries which supply the heart with blood are the first vessels given off from the great feeding arterial trunk, and the veins of the heart winding independently round it empty their contents direct again into it. Thus is the heart the most perfect of independencies: thus during sleep and during wakefulness it works its own course, and, taking first care of itself in every particular, feeds the rest of the body afterward; thus, even when sleep passes into death, the heart in almost every case continues its action for some time after all the other parts of the organism are in absolute quiescence; thus, in hibernating animals, the heart continues in play during their long somnolence; and, thus, under the insensibility produced by the inhalation of narcotic gases and vapors, the heart sustains its function when every other part is temporarily dead. Next the heart in independent action is the muscle called the midriff or diaphragm; and, as the diaphragm is a muscle of inspiration, the respiratory function plays second to the circulatory, and the two great functions of life are, in sleep, faithfully performed. In sleep of illness bordering on sleep of death, how intently we watch for the merest trace of breath, and augur that, if but a feather be moved by it or a mirror dimmed by it, there is yet life!

In natural sleep, then, sleep perfect and deep, that half of our nature which is volitional is in the condition of inertia. To say, as Blumenbach has said, that in this state all intercourse between mind and body is suspended, is more perhaps than should be said, the precise limits and connections of mind and body being unknown. But certainly the brain and spinal cord, ceasing themselves to receive impressions, cease to communicate to the muscles they supply stimulus for motion, and the muscles under their control, with their nerves, therefore sleep. And so, to the extent that the acts of the brain and cord and their nerves are mental, and the acts or motions of the voluntary muscles are bodily acts, to that extent, in sleep, the intercourse between the mind and the body is suspended.

In sleep the condition of the involuntary muscles and of the voluntary nervous system is, we must assume, in some manner modified, since these organs are transformed from the active into the passive state. Respecting the condition of the muscles in sleep, no study of a systematic sort has been carried out, but in relation to the brain there has been much thoughtful study, upon which many theories have been founded.

The older physiologists regarded sleep as due to the exhaustion of the nervous fluid; during sleep, they held, this fluid accumulates in the brain; and, when the brain and the other centers and nerves of the cerebro-spinal system are, to employ a common expression, recharged, the muscles are stimulated and the body awakes; the brain prepared to receive external impressions and to animate the muscles, and the muscles renovated and ready to be recalled into activity. This theory held its ground for many years, and, perhaps, still there are more believers in it than in any other. It fails to convince the skeptical because of its incompleteness, for it tells nothing about the nature of the presumed nervous fluid, and we know nothing as yet about this fluid. The primary step of the speculation is consequently itself purely hypothetical.

Another theory, that has been promulgated, is that sleep depends on the sinking or collapse of the laminæ of the cerebellum or little brain. This theory is based on the experiment that compression of the cerebellum induces sleep; but the argument is fallacious, because pressure on the larger brain, or cerebrum, is followed by the same result. The theory of pressure has been proposed again in a different way; it has been affirmed that the phenomenon of sleep is caused by the accumulation of fluids in the cavity of the cranium, and by pressure, resulting from this accumulation, on the brain as a whole. We know well that pressure upon the brain does lead to an insensible condition resembling sleep, and in some instances, in which the skull has been injured and an artificial opening through it to the brain has been formed, pressure upon the exposed surface has led to a comatose condition. I once myself saw a case of this nature. But the evidence against this explanation is strong, because the sleeping brain has been observed to be pale and too free of blood to convey any idea of pressure.

In opposition to the pressure theory, Blumenbach contended that sleep is due to a diminished flow and impulse of blood upon the brain, for he argued the phenomenon of sleep is induced by exhaustion, and particularly by exhaustion following upon direct loss of blood. Recently Mr. Arthur Durham, in a very able communication, has adduced a similar view, and the general conclusion now is, that during sleep the brain is really supplied with less blood than in waking hours.

To account for the reason why the brain is less freely fed with blood in sleep, it has been surmised that the vessels, the arteries, which feed the brain, and which for contractile purposes are supplied with nerves from the organic nervous system, are, under their nervous influence, made to close so that a portion at least of the blood which enters through them is cut off on going to sleep. This view, however, presupposes that the organic nervous centers, instead of sharing in the exhaustion incident to labor, put forth increased power after fatigue, an idea incompatible with all we know of the natural functions.

Carmichael, an excellent physiologist, thought that sleep was brought on by a change in the assimilation of the brain, and by what he called the deposition of new matter in the organ, but he offered no evidence in proof: while Metcalfe, one of the most learned physicists and physicians of our time, maintained that the proximate cause of sleep is an expenditure of the substance and vital energy of the brain, nerves, and voluntary muscles, beyond what they receive when awake, and that the specific office of sleep is the restoration of what has been wasted by exercise: the most remarkable difference between exercise and sleep being, that during exercise the expenditure exceeds the income; whereas during sleep the income exceeds the expenditure. This idea of Metcalfe's expresses, probably, a broad truth, but it is too general to indicate the proximate cause of sleep, to explain which is the object of his proposition.

My own researches on the proximate cause of sleep—researches which of late years have been steadily pursued—lead me to the conclusion that none of the theories as yet offered account correctly for the natural phenomenon of sleep; although I must express that some of them are based on well-defined facts. It is perfectly true that exhaustion of the brain will induce phenomena so closely allied to the phenomena of natural sleep, that no one could tell the artificially-induced from the natural sleep; and it is equally true that pressure upon the brain will also lead to a state of sleep simulating the natural. For example, in a young animal, a pigeon, I can induce the deepest sleep by exposing the brain to the influence of extreme cold. I have had a bird sleeping calmly for ten hours under the local influence of cold. During this time the state of the brain is one of extreme blood lessness, and, when the cold is cautiously withdrawn and the brain is allowed to refill gently with blood, the sleep passes away. This is clear enough, and the cold, it may be urged, produces contraction of the brain-substance and of the vessels, with diminution of blood, and with sleep as the result. But if, when the animal is awaking from this sleep induced by cold, I apply warmth, for the unsealing of the parts, a little too freely, if, that is to say, I restore the natural warmth too quickly, then the animal falls asleep again under an opposite condition; for now into the relaxed vessels of the brain the heart injects blood so freely, that the vessels, in like manner as when the frozen hand is held near the fire, become engorged with blood, there is congestion, there is pressure, and there is sleep.

The same series of phenomena from opposite conditions can be induced by narcotic vapors. There is a fluid called chloride of aonyl, which, by inhalation, causes the deepest sleep; during the sleep so induced, the brain is as bloodless as if it were frozen. There is an ether called methylic, which, by inhalation, can be made to produce the deepest sleep; during this sleep the vessels of the brain are engorged with blood.

We are therefore correct in supposing that artificial sleep may be induced both by removal of blood from the brain, and by pressure of blood upon the brain; and in the facts there is, when we consider them, nothing extraordinary. In both conditions, the natural state of the brain is altered; it cannot, under either state, properly receive or transmit motion; so it is quiescent, it sleeps. The experimental proof of this can be performed on any part of the body where there are nerve-fibre and blood-vessel; if I freeze a portion of my skin, by ether-spray, I make it insensible to all impression—I make it sleep; if I place over a portion of skin a cupping-tube, and forcibly induce intense congestion of vessels, by exhausting the air of the tube, I make the part also insensible—I make it sleep.

The two most plausible theories of sleep—the plenum and the vacuum theories I had nearly called them—are, then, based on facts; but still I think them fallacious. The theory that natural sleep depends on pressure of the brain from blood is disproved by the observations that have been made of the brain during sleep, while the mechanism of the circulation through the brain furnishes no thought of this theory as being possibly correct. The theory that sleep is caused by withdrawal of blood from the brain, by contraction of its arterial vessels, is disproved by many considerations. It presupposes that at the time when the cerebrospinal nervous system is most wearied the organic system is most active; and it assumes that the great volume of blood which circulates through the brain can be cut off without evidence of increased volume of blood and tension of vessel in other parts of the body, a supposition directly negatived by the actual experiment of cutting off the blood from the brain.

There is another potent objection applicable to both theories. When sleep is artificially induced, either by subjecting the brain to pressure of blood, or to exhaustion of blood, the sleep is of such a kind that the sleeper cannot be roused until the influence at work to produce the sleep is removed. But, in natural sleep, the sleeper can always be roused by motion or vibration. We call to a person supposed to be sleeping naturally, or we shake him, and if we cannot rouse him we know there is danger; but how could these simple acts remove pressure from the brain, or relax the contracted vessels feeding the brain?

These two theories set aside, the others I have named need not trouble us; they are mere generalizations, interesting to read, worthless to pursue. Know we then nothing leading toward a solution of the question of the proximate cause of sleep? I cannot say that, for I think we see our way to something which will unravel the phenomenon; but we must work slowly and patiently, and as men assured that, in the problem we are endeavoring to solve, we are dealing with a subject of more than ordinary importance. I will try to point out the direction of research.

I find that to induce sleep it is not necessary to produce extreme changes of brain-matter. In applying cold, for example, it is not necessary to make the brain-substance solid in order to induce stupor, but simply to bring down its temperature ten or twelve degrees. I find also that very slight direct vibrations, concussions, will induce stupor; and I find that, in animals of different kinds, the profoundness of sleep is greater in proportion as the size of the brain is larger. From these and other facts, I infer that the phenomenon of natural sleep is due to a molecular change in the nervous structure itself of the cerebro-spinal system, and that in *perfect* sleep the whole of the nervous structure is involved in the change—the brain, the cord, the nerves; while in imperfect sleep only parts of this nervous matter are influenced. This is in accord with facts, for I can by cold put to sleep special parts of the nervous mass without putting other parts to sleep. In bad sleep we have the representation of the same thing in the restlessness of the muscles, the half-conscious wakings, the dreams.

Suppose this idea of the change of nervous matter to be true, is there any clew to the nature of the change itself? I think there is. The change is one very closely resembling that which occurs in the solidification of water surcharged with a saline substance, or in water holding a hydrated colloid, like dialyzed silica, in trembling suspension. What is, indeed, the brain and nervous matter? It is a mass of water made sufficiently solid to be reduced into shape and form, by rather less than twenty per cent, of solid matter, consisting of albuminous substance, saline substance, fatty substance. The mechanism for the supply of blood is most delicate, membranous; the mechanism for dialysis or separation of crystalloidal from colloidal substance is perfect, and the conversion of the compound substance of brain from one condition of matter to another is, if we may judge from some changes of water charged with colloidal or fatty substances, extremely simple. I do not now venture on details respecting this peculiarly interesting question, but I venture so far as to express what I feel will one day be the accepted fact, that the matter of the wakeful brain is, on going to sleep, changed, temporarily, into a state of greater solidity; that its molecular parts cease to be moved by external ordinary influences, by chemical influences; that they, in turn, cease to communicate impressions, or, in other words, to stimulate the voluntary muscles; and that then there is sleep which lasts until there is resolution of structure, whereupon there is wakefulness, from renewed motion in brain-matter, and renewed stimulation of voluntary muscle, through nerve.

The change of structure of the brain which I assume to be the proximate cause of sleep is possibly the same change as occurs in a more extreme degree when the brain and its subordinate parts actually die. The effects of a concussion of the brain from a blow, the effects of a simple puncture of nervous matter in centers essential to life—as the point in the medulla oblongata which Flourens has designated the vital point—have never been explained, and admit, I imagine, of no explanation except the change of structure I have now ventured to suggest.

Here, for the moment, my task must end. My object has been to make the reader conversant with what has been said by philosophers upon the subject of sleep and its proximate cause, and to indicate briefly a new Line of scientific inquiry. I shall hope on some future occasion to be able to announce further and more fruitful labor.

The Laws of Sleep[3]

Definition of sleep.

The following are the characteristic circumstances attending perfect sleep.

1. The power of volition is totally suspended.

2. The trains of ideas caused by sensation proceed with greater facility and vivacity; but become inconsistent with the usual order of nature. The muscular motions caused by sensation continue; as those concerned in our evacuations during infancy, and afterwards in digestion, and in priapismus.

3. The irritative muscular motions continue, as those concerned in the circulation, in secretion, in respiration. But the irritative sensual motions, or ideas, are not excited; as the immediate organs of sense are not stimulated into action by external objects, which are excluded by the external organs of sense; which

---

[3] by Erasmus Darwin.

are not in sleep adapted to their reception by the power of volition, as in our waking hours.

4. The associate motions continue; but their first link is not excited into action by volition, or by external stimuli. In all respects, except those above mentioned, the three last sensorial powers are somewhat increased in energy during the suspension of volition, owing to the consequent accumulation of the spirit of animation.

1. *Volition is suspended in sleep.*

There are four situations of our system, which in their moderate degrees are not usually termed diseases, and yet abound with many very curious and instructive phenomena; these are sleep, reverie, vertigo, drunkenness. These we shall previously consider, before we step forwards to develop the causes and cures of diseases with the modes of the operation of medicines.

As all those trains and tribes of animal motion, which are subjected to volition, were the last that were caused, their connection is weaker than that of the other classes; and there is a peculiar circumstance attending this causation, which is, that it is entirely suspended during sleep; whilst the other classes of motion, which are more immediately necessary to life, as those caused by internal stimuli, for instance the pulsations of the heart and arteries, or those catenated with pleasurable sensation, as the powers of digestion, continue to strengthen their habits without interruption. Thus though man in his sleeping state is a much less perfect animal, than in his waking hours; and though he consumes more than one third of his life in this his irrational situation; yet is the wisdom of the Author of nature manifest even in this seeming imperfection of his work!

The truth of this assertion with respect to the large muscles of the body, which are concerned in locomotion, is evident; as no one in perfect sanity walks about in his sleep, or performs any domestic offices: and in respect to the mind, we never exercise our reason or recollection in dreams; we may sometimes seem distracted between contending passions, but we never compare their objects, or deliberate about the acquisition of those objects, if our sleep is perfect. And though many synchronous tribes or successive trains of ideas may represent the houses or walks, which have real existence, yet are they here introduced by their connection with our sensations, and are in truth ideas of imagination, not of recollection.

2. *Sensation continues. Dreams prevent delirium and inflammation.*

For our sensations of pleasure and pain are experienced with great vivacity in our dreams; and hence all that motley group of ideas, which are caused by them, called the ideas of imagination, with their various associated trains, are in a very vivid manner acted over in the sensorium; and these sometimes call into action the larger muscles, which have been much associated with them; as appears from the muttering sentences, which some people utter in their dreams, and from the obscure barking of sleeping dogs, and the motions of their feet and nostrils.

This perpetual flow of the trains of ideas, which constitute our dreams, and which are caused by painful or pleasurable sensation, might at first view be conceived to be an useless expenditure of sensorial power. But it has been shewn, that those motions, which are perpetually excited, as those of the arterial system by the stimulus of the blood, are attended by a great accumulation of sensorial power, after they have been for a time suspended; as the hot-fit of fever is the consequence of the cold one. Now as these trains of ideas caused by sensation are perpetually excited during our waking hours, if they were to be suspended in sleep like the voluntary motions, (which are exerted only by intervals during our waking hours,) an accumulation of sensorial power would follow; and on our awaking a delirium would supervene, since these ideas caused by sensation would be produced with such energy, that we should mistake the trains of imagination for ideas excited by irritation; as perpetually happens to people debilitated by fevers on their first awaking; for in these fevers with debility the general quantity of irritation being diminished, that of sensation is increased. In like manner if the actions of the stomach, intestines, and various glands, which are perhaps in part at least caused by or catenated with agreeable sensation, and which perpetually exist during our waking hours, were like the voluntary motions suspended in our sleep; the great accumulation of sensorial power, which would necessarily follow, would be liable to excite inflammation in them.

3. *Nightmare.*

When by our continued posture in sleep, some uneasy sensations are produced, we either gradually awake by the exertion of volition, or the muscles connected by habit with such sensations alter the position of the body; but where the sleep is uncommonly profound, and those uneasy sensations great, the disease called the incubus, or nightmare, is produced. Here the desire of moving the body is painfully exerted, by the power of moving it, or volition, is incapable of action, till we awake. Many less disagreeable struggles in our dreams, as when we wish in vain to fly from terrifying objects, constitute a slighter degree of this disease. In awaking from the nightmare I have more than once observed, that there was no disorder in my pulse; nor do I believe the respiration is laborious, as some have affirmed. It occurs to people whose sleep is too profound, and some disagreeable sensation exists, which at other times would have awakened them, and have thence prevented the disease of nightmare; as after great fatigue or hunger with too large a supper and wine, which occasion our sleep to be uncommonly profound. See N°. 14, of this Section.

4. *Ceaseless flow of ideas in dreams.*

As the larger muscles of the body are much more frequently excited by volition than by sensation, they are but seldom brought into action in our sleep: but the ideas of the mind are by habit much more frequently connected with sensation than with volition; and hence the ceaseless flow of our ideas in dreams. Every one's experience will teach him this truth, for we all daily exert much voluntary muscular motion: but few of mankind can bear the fatigue of much voluntary thinking.

5. *We seem to receive them by the senses. Optic nerve perfectly sensible in sleep. Eyes less dazzled after dreaming of visible objects.*

A very curious circumstance attending these our sleeping imaginations is, that we seem to receive them by the senses. The muscles, which are subservient to the external organs of sense, are connected with volition, and cease to act in sleep; hence the eyelids are closed, and the tympanum of the ear relaxed; and it is probable a similarity of voluntary exertion may be necessary for the perceptions of the other nerves of sense; for it is observed that the papillæ of the tongue can be seen to become erected, when we attempt to taste anything extremely grateful. Add to this, that the immediate organs of sense have no objects to excite them in the darkness and silence of the night, but their nerves of sense nevertheless continue to possess their perfect activity subservient to all their numerous sensitive connections. This vivacity of our nerves of sense during the time of sleep is evinced by a circumstance, which almost every one must at some time or other have experienced; that is, if we sleep in the daylight, and endeavour to see some object in our dream, the light is exceedingly painful to our eyes; and after repeated struggles we lament in our sleep, that we cannot see it. In this case I apprehend the eyelid is in some degree opened by the vehemence of our sensations; and, the iris being dilated, the optic nerve shews as great or greater sensibility than in our waking hours. See Nº15 of this Section.

When we are forcibly waked at midnight from profound sleep, our eyes are much dazzled with the light of the candle for a minute or two, after there has been sufficient time allowed for the contraction of the iris; which is owing to the accumulation of sensorial power in the organ of vision during its state of less activity. But when we have dreamt much of visible objects, this accumulation of sensorial power in the organ of vision is lessened or prevented, and we awake in the morning without being dazzled with the light, after the iris has had time to contract itself. This is a matter of great curiosity, and may be thus tried by any one in the day-light. Close your eyes, and cover them with your hat; think for a minute on a tune, which you are accustomed to, and endeavour to sing it with as little activity of mind as possible. Suddenly uncover and open your eyes, and in one second of time the iris will contract itself, but you will perceive the day more luminous for several seconds, owing to the accumulation of sensorial power in the optic nerve.

Then again close and cover your eyes, and think intensely on a cube of ivory two inches diameter, attending first to the north and south sides of it, and then to the other four sides of it; then get a clear image in your mind's eye of all the sides of the same cube coloured red; and then of it coloured green; and then of it coloured blue; lastly, open your eyes as in the former experiment, and after the first second of time allowed for the contraction of the iris, you will not perceive any increase of the light of the day, or dazzling; because now there is no accumulation of sensorial power in the optic nerve; that having been expended by its action in thinking over visible objects.

This experiment is not easy to be made at first, but by a few patient trials the fact appears very certain; and shows clearly, that our ideas of imagination are repetitions of the motions of the nerve, which were originally occasioned by the stimulus of external bodies; because they equally expend the sensorial power in the organ of sense. which is analogous to our being as much fatigued by thinking as by labour.

6. *Reverie, belief.*

Nor is it in our dreams alone, but even in our waking reveries, and in great efforts of invention, so great is the vivacity of our ideas, that we do not for a time distinguish them from the real presence of substantial objects; though the external organs of sense are open, and surrounded with their usual stimuli. Thus whilst I am thinking over the beautiful valley, through which I yesterday travelled, I do not perceive the furniture of my room: and there are some, whose waking imaginations are so apt to run into perfect reverie, that in their common attention to a favourite idea they do not hear the voice of the companion, who accosts them, unless it is repeated with unusual energy.

This perpetual mistake in dreams and reveries, where our ideas of imagination are attended with a belief of the presence of external objects, evinces beyond a doubt, that all our ideas are repetitions of the motions of the nerves of sense, by which they were acquired; and that this belief is not, as some late philosophers contend, an instinct necessarily connected only with our perceptions.

7. *How we distinguish ideas from perceptions.*

A curious question demands our attention in this place; as we do not distinguish in our dreams and reveries between our perceptions of external objects, and our ideas of them in their absence, how do we distinguish them at any time? In a dream, if the sweetness of sugar occurs to my imagination, the whiteness and hardness of it, which were ideas usually connected with the sweetness, immediately follow in the train; and I believe a material lump of sugar present before my senses: but in my waking hours, if the sweetness occurs to my imagination, the stimulus of the table to my hand, or of the window to my eye, prevents the other ideas of the hardness and whiteness of the sugar from succeeding; and hence I perceive the fallacy, and disbelieve the existence of objects correspondent to those ideas, whose tribes or trains are broken by the stimulus of other objects. And further in our waking hours, we frequently exert our volition in comparing present appearances with such, as we have usually observed; and thus correct the errors of one sense by our general knowledge of nature by intuitive analogy. Whereas in dreams the power of volition is suspended, we can recollect and compare our present ideas with none of our acquired knowledge, and are hence incapable of observing any absurdities in them.

By this criterion we distinguish our waking from our sleeping hours, we can voluntarily recollect our sleeping ideas, when we are awake, and compare them with our waking ones; but we cannot in our sleep *voluntarily* recollect our waking ideas at all.

8. *Variety of scenery in dreams, excellence of the sense of vision.*

The vast variety of scenery, novelty of combination, and distinctness of imagery, are other curious circumstances of our sleeping imaginations. The variety of scenery seems to arise from the superior activity and excellence of our sense of vision; which in an instant unfolds to the mind extensive fields of pleasurable ideas; while the other senses collect their objects slowly, and with little combination; add to this, that the ideas, which this organ presents us with, are more frequently connected with our sensation than those of any other.

9. *Novelty of combination in dreams.*

The great novelty of combination is owing to another circumstance; the trains of ideas, which are carried on in our waking thoughts, are in our dreams dissevered in a thousand places by the suspension of volition, and the absence of irritative ideas, and are hence perpetually falling into new catenations. For the power of volition is perpetually exerted during our waking hours in comparing our passing trains of ideas with our acquired knowledge of nature, and thus forms many intermediate links in their catenation. And the irritative ideas excited by the stimulus of the objects, with which we are surrounded, are every moment intruded upon us, and form other links of our unceasing catenations of ideas.

10. *Distinctness of imagery in dreams.*

The absence of the stimuli of external bodies, and of volition, in our dreams renders the organs of sense liable to be more strongly affected by the powers of sensation, and of association. For our desires or aversions, or the obtrusions of surrounding bodies, dissever the sensitive and associate tribes of ideas in our waking hours by introducing those of irritation and volition amongst them. Hence proceeds the superior distinctness of pleasurable or painful imagery in our sleep; for we recal the figure and the features of a long lost friend, whom we loved, in our dreams with much more accuracy and vivacity than in our waking thoughts. This circumstance contributes to prove, that our ideas of imagination are reiterations of those motions of our organs of sense, which were excited by external objects; because while we are exposed to the stimuli of present objects, our ideas of absent objects cannot be so distinctly formed.

11. *Rapidity of transaction in dreams.*

The rapidity of the succession of transactions in our dreams is almost inconceivable; insomuch that, when we are accidentally awakened by the jarring of a door, which is opened into our bed-chamber, we sometimes dream a whole history of thieves or fire in the very instant of awaking.

During the suspension of volition we cannot compare our other ideas with those of the parts of time in which they exist; that is, we cannot compare the imaginary scene, which is before us, with those changes of it, which precede or follow it: because this act of comparing requires recollection or voluntary exertion. Whereas in our waking hours, we are perpetually making this comparison, and by that means our waking ideas are kept confident with each other by intuitive analogy; but this companion retards the succession of them, by occasioning their repetition. Add to this, that the transactions of our dreams consist chiefly of visible ideas, and that a whole history of thieves and fire may be *beheld* in an instant of time like the figures in a picture.

12. *Of measuring time. Of dramatic time and place. Why a dull play induces sleep, and an interesting one reverie.*

From this incapacity of attending to the parts of time in our dreams, arises our ignorance of the length of the night; which, but from our constant experience to the contrary, we should conclude was but a few minutes, when our sleep is perfect. The same happens in our reveries; thus when we are possessed with vehement joy, grief, or anger, time appears short, for we exert no volition to compare the present scenery with the past or future; but when we are compelled to perform those exercises of mind or body, which, are unmixed with passion, as in travelling over a dreary country, time appears long; for our desire to finish our journey occasions us more frequently to compare our present situation with the parts of time or place, which are before and behind us.

So when we are enveloped in deep contemplation of any kind, or in reverie, as in reading a very interesting play or romance, we measure time very inaccurately; and hence, if a play greatly affects our passions, the absurdities of passing over many days or years, and or perpetual changes of place, are not perceived by the audience; as is experienced by everyone, who reads or sees some plays of the immortal Shakespeare; but it is necessary for inferior authors to observe those rules of the πιθανον and πρεπον inculcated by Aristotle, because their works do not interest the passions sufficiently to produce complete reverie.

Those works, however, whether a romance or a sermon, which do not interest us so much as to induce reverie, may nevertheless incline us to sleep. For those pleasurable ideas, which are presented to us, and are too gentle to excite laughter, (which is attended with interrupted voluntary exertions, and which are not accompanied with any other emotion, which usually excites some voluntary exertion, as anger, or fear, are liable to produce sleep; which consists in a suspension of all voluntary power. But if the ideas thus presented to us, and interest our attention, are accompanied with so much pleasurable or painful sensation as to excite our voluntary exertion at the same time, reverie is the consequence. Hence an interesting play produces reverie, a tedious one produces sleep: in the latter we become exhausted by attention, and are not excited to any voluntary exertion, and therefore sleep; in the former we are excited by some emotion, which prevents by its pain the suspension of volition, and in as much as it interests us, induces reverie, as explained in the next Section.

But when our sleep is imperfect, as when we have determined to rise in half an hour, time appears longer to us than in most other situations. Here our solicitude not to oversleep the determined time induces us in this imperfect sleep to compare the quick changes of imagined scenery with the parts of time or place, they would have taken up, had they real exigence; and that more frequently than in our waking hours; and hence the time appears longer to us: and I make no doubt, but the permitted time appears long to a man going to the gallows, as the fear of its quick lapse will make him think frequently about it.

13. *Consciousness of our existence and identity in dreams.*

As we gain our knowledge of time by comparing the present scenery with the past and future, and of place by comparing the situations of objects with each other; so we gain our idea of consciousness by comparing ourselves with the scenery around us; and of identity by comparing our present consciousness with our past consciousness: as we never think of time or place, but when we make the companions above mentioned, so we never think of consciousness, but when we compare our own existence with that of other objects; nor of identity, but when we compare our present and our past consciousness. Hence the consciousness of our own existence, and of our identity, is owing to a voluntary exertion of our minds: and on that account in our complete dreams we neither measure time, are surprised at the sudden changes of place, nor attend to our own existence, or identity; because our power of volition is suspended. But all these circumstances are more or less observable in our incomplete ones; for then we attend a little to the lapse of time, and the changes of place, and to our own existence; and even to our identity of person; for a lady seldom dreams, that she is a soldier; nor a man, that he is brought to bed.

14. *How we awake sometimes suddenly, sometimes frequently.*

As long as our sensations only excite their sensual motions, or ideas, our sleep continues sound; but as soon as they excite desires or aversions, our sleep becomes imperfect; and when that desire or aversion is so strong, as to produce voluntary motions, we begin to awake; the larger muscles of the body are brought into action to remove that irritation or sensation, which a continued posture has caused; we stretch our limbs, and yawn, and our sleep is thus broken by the accumulation of voluntary power.

Sometimes it happens, that the act of waking is suddenly produced, and this soon after the commencement of sleep; which is occasioned by some sensation so disagreeable, as instantaneously to excite the power of volition; and a temporary action of all the voluntary motions suddenly succeeds, and we start awake. This is sometimes accompanied with loud noise in the ears, and with some degree of fear; and when it is in great excess, so as to produce continued convulsive motions of those muscles, which are generally subservient to volition, it becomes epilepsy: the fits of which in some patients generally commence during sleep. This differs from the nightmare described in N° 3. of this Section, because in that the disagreeable sensation is not so great as to excite the power of volition into action; for as soon as that happens, the disease ceases.

Another circumstance, which sometimes awakes people soon after the commencement of their sleep, is where the voluntary power is already so great in quantity as almost to prevent them from falling asleep, and then a little accumulation of it soon again awakens them; this happens in cases of insanity, or where the mind has been lately much agitated by fear or anger. There is another circumstance in which sleep is likewise of short duration, which arises from great debility, as after great over-fatigue, and in some fevers, where the strength of the patient is greatly diminished, as in these cases the pulse intermits or flutters, and the respiration is previously affected, it seems to originate from the want of some voluntary efforts to facilitate respiration, as when we are awake.

15. *Why we feel chilly at the approach of sleep, and at waking in the open air.*

We come now to those motions which depend on irritation. The motions of the arterial and glandular systems continue in our sleep, proceeding slower indeed, but stronger and more uniformly, than in our waking hours, when they are incommoded by external stimuli, or by the movements of volition; the motions of the muscles subservient to respiration continue to be stimulated into action, and the other internal senses of hunger, thirst, and lust, are not only occasionally excited in our sleep, but their irritative motions are succeeded by their usual sensations, and make a part of the farrago of our dreams. These sensations of the want of air, of hunger, thirst, and lust, in our dreams, contribute to prove, that the nerves of the external senses are also alive and excitable in our sleep; but as the stimuli of external objects are either excluded from them by the darkness and silence of the night, or their access to them is prevented by the suspension of volition, these nerves of sense fall more readily into their connexions with sensation and with association; because much sensorial power, which during the day was expended in moving the external organs of sense in consequence of irritation from external stimuli, or in consequence of volition, becomes now in some degree accumulated, and renders the internal or immediate organs of sense more easily excitable by the other sensorial powers. Thus in respect to the eye, the irritation from external stimuli, and the power of volition during our waking hours, elevate the eye-lids, adapt the aperture of the iris to the quantity of light, the focus of the crystalline humour, and the angle of the optic axises to the distance of the object, all which perpetual activity during the day expends much sensorial power, which is saved during our sleep.

Hence it appears, that not only those parts of the system, which are always excited by internal stimuli, as the stomach, intestinal canal, bile-ducts, and the various glands, but the organs of sense also may be more violently excited into action by the irritation from internal stimuli, or by sensation, during our sleep than in our waking hours; because during the suspension of volition, there is a greater quantity of the spirit of animation to be expended by the other sensorial powers. On this account our irritability to internal stimuli, and our sensibility to pain or pleasure, is not only greater in sleep, but increases as our sleep is prolonged. Whence digestion and secretion are performed better in sleep, than in our waking hours, and our dreams in the morning have greater variety and vivacity, as our sensibility increases, than at night when we first lie down. And hence epileptic fits, which are always occasioned by some disagreeable sensation, so frequently attack those, who are subject to them, in their sleep; because at this time the system is more excitable by painful sensation in consequence of internal stimuli; and the power of volition is then suddenly exerted to relieve this pain.

There is a disease, which frequently affects children in the cradle, which is termed ecstasy, and seems to consist in certain exertions to relieve painful sensation, in which the voluntary power is not so far excited as totally to awaken them, and yet is sufficient to remove the disagreeable sensation, which excites it; in this case changing the posture of the child frequently relieves it.

I have at this time under my care an elegant young man about twenty-two years of age, who seldom sleeps more than an hour without experiencing a convulsion fit; which ceases in about half a minute without any subsequent stupor. Large doses of opium only prevented the paroxysms, so long as they prevented him from sleeping by the intoxication, which they induced. Other medicines had no effect on him. He was gently awakened every half hour for one night, but without good effect, as he soon slept again, and the fit returned at about the same periods of time, for the accumulated sensorial power, which occasioned the increased sensibility to pain, was not thus exhausted. This case evinces, that the sensibility of the system to internal excitation increases, as our sleep is prolonged; till the pain thus occasioned produces voluntary exertion; which, when it is in its usual degree, only awakens us; but when it is more violent, it occasions convulsions.

The cramp in the calf of the leg is another kind of convulsion, which generally commences in sleep, occasioned by the continual increase of irritability from internal stimuli, or of sensibility, during that state of our existence. The cramp is a violent exertion to relieve pain, generally either of the skin from cold, or of the bowels, as in some diarrhœas, or from the muscles having been previously overstretched, as in walking up or down steep hills. But in these convulsions of the muscles, which form the calf of the leg, the contraction is so violent as to occasion another pain in consequence of their own too violent contraction; as soon as the original pain, which caused the contraction, is removed. And hence the cramp, or spasm, of these muscles is continued without intermission by this new pain, unlike the alternate convulsions and remissions in epileptic fits. The reason, that the contraction of these muscles of the calf of the leg is more violent during their convulsion than that of others, depends on the weakness of their antagonist muscles; for after these have been contracted in their usual action, as at every step in walking, they are again extended, not, as most other muscles are, by their antagonists, but by the weight of the whole body on the balls of the toes; and that weight applied to great mechanical advantage on the heel, that is, on the other end of the bone of the foot, which thus acts as a lever.

Another disease, the periods of which generally commence during our sleep, is the asthma. Whatever may be the remote cause of paroxysms of asthma, the immediate cause of the convulsive respiration, whether in the common asthma, or in what is termed the convulsive asthma, which are perhaps only different degrees of the same disease, must be owing to violent voluntary exertions to relieve pain, as in other convulsions; and the increase of irritability to internal stimuli, or of sensibility, during sleep must occasion them to commence at this time.

Debilitated people, who have been unfortunately accustomed to great ingurgitation of spirituous potation, frequently part with a great quantity of water during the night, but with not more than usual in the day-time. This is owing to a beginning torpor of the absorbent system, and precedes anasarca, which commences in the day, but is cured in the night by the increase of the irritability of the absorbent system during sleep, which thus imbibes from the cellular membrane the fluids, which had been accumulated there during the day; though it is possible the horizontal position of the body may contribute something to this purpose, and also the greater irritability of some branches of the absorbent vessels, which open their mouths in the cells of the cellular membrane, than that of other branches.

As soon as a person begins to sleep, the irritability and sensibility of the system begins to increase, owing to the suspension of volition and the exclusion of external stimuli. Hence the actions of the vessels in obedience to internal stimulation become stronger and more energetic, though less frequent in respect to number. And as many of the secretions are increased, so the heat of the system is gradually increased, and the extremities of feeble people, which had been cold during the day, become warm. Till towards morning many people become so warm, as to find it necessary to throw off some of their bed-clothes, as soon as they awake; and in others sweats are so liable to occur towards morning during their sleep.

Thus those, who are not accustomed to sleep in the open air, are very liable to take cold, if they happen to fall asleep on a garden bench, or in a carriage with the window open. For as the system is warmer during sleep, as above explained, if a current of cold air affects any part of the body, a torpor of that part is more effectually produced, as when a cold blast of air through a key-hole or casement falls upon a person in a warm room. In those cases the affected part possesses less irritability in respect to heat, from its having previously been exposed to a greater stimulus of heat, as in the warm room, or during sleep; and hence, when the stimulus of heat is diminished, a torpor is liable to ensue; that is, we take cold. Hence people who sleep in the open air, generally feel chilly both at the approach of sleep, and on their awaking; and hence many people are perpetually subject to catarrhs if they sleep in a less warm head-dress, than that which they wear in the day.

16. *Why the gout commences in sleep. Secretions are more copious in sleep, young animals and plants grow more in sleep.*

Not only the sensorial powers of irritation and of sensation, but that of association also appear to act with greater vigour during the suspension of volition in sleep. It will be shown in another place, that the gout generally first attacks the liver, and that afterwards an inflammation of the ball of the great toe commences by association, and that of the liver ceases. Now as this change or metastasis of the activity of the system generally commences in sleep, it follows, that these associations of motion exist with greater energy at that time; that is, that the sensorial faculty of association, like those of irritation and of sensation, becomes in some measure accumulated during the suspension of volition.

Other associate tribes and trains of motions, as well as the irritative and sensitive ones, appear to be increased in their activity during the suspension of volition in sleep. As those which contribute to circulate the blood, and to perform the various secretions; as well as the associate tribes and trains of ideas, which contribute to furnish the perpetual dreams of our dreaming imaginations.

In sleep the secretions have generally been supposed to be diminished, as the expectorated mucus in coughs, the fluids discharged in diarrhœas, and in salivation, except indeed the secretion of sweat, which is often visibly increased. This error seems to have arisen from attention to the excretions rather than to the secretions. For the secretions, except that of sweat, are generally received into reservoirs, as the urine into the bladder, and the mucus of the intestines and lungs into their respective cavities; but these reservoirs do not exclude these fluids immediately by their stimulus, but require at the same time some voluntary efforts, and therefore permit them to remain during sleep. And as they thus continue longer in those receptacles in our sleeping hours, a greater part is absorbed from them, and the remainder becomes thicker, and sometimes in less quantity, though at the time it was secreted the fluid was in greater quantity than in our waking hours. Thus the urine is higher coloured after long sleep; which shows that a greater quantity has been secreted, and that more of the aqueous and saline part has been reabsorbed, and the earthy part left in the bladder; hence thick urine in fevers shows only a greater action of the vessels which secrete it in the kidneys, and of those which absorb it from the bladder.

The same happens to the mucus expectorated in coughs, which is thus thickened by absorption of its aqueous and saline parts; and the same of the feces of the intestines. From hence it appears, and from what has been said in N° 15. of this Section concerning the increase of irritability and of sensibility during sleep, that the secretions are in general rather increased than diminished during these hours of our existence; and it is probable that nutrition is almost entirely performed in sleep; and that young animals grow more at this time than in their waking hours, as young plants have long since been observed to grow more in the night, which is their time of sleep.

17. _Inconsistency of dreams. Absence of surprise in dreams._

Two other remarkable circumstances of our dreaming ideas are their inconsistency, and the total absence of surprise. Thus we seem to be present at more extraordinary metamorphoses of animals or trees, than are to be met with in the fables of antiquity; and appear to be transported from place to place, which seas divide, as quickly as the changes of scenery are performed in a play-house; and yet are not sensible of their inconsistency, nor in the least degree affected with surprise.

We must consider this circumstance more minutely. In our waking trains of ideas, those that are inconsistent with the usual order of nature, so rarely have occurred to us, that their connexion is the slightest of all others: hence, when a consistent train of ideas is exhausted, we attend to the external stimuli, that usually surround us, rather than to any inconsistent idea, which might otherwise present itself; and if an inconsistent idea should intrude itself, we immediately compare it with the preceding one, and voluntarily reject the train it would introduce; this appears further in the Section on Reverie, in which state of the mind external stimuli are not attended to, and yet the streams of ideas are kept consistent by the efforts of volition. But as our faculty of volition is suspended, and all external stimuli are excluded in sleep, this slighter connexion of ideas takes place; and the train is said to be inconsistent; that is, dissimilar to the usual order of nature.

But, when any consistent train of sensitive or voluntary ideas is flowing along, if any external stimulus affects us so violently, as to intrude irritative ideas forcibly into the mind, it disunites the former train of ideas, and we are affected with surprise. These stimuli of unusual energy or novelty not only disunite our common trains of ideas, but the trains of muscular motions also, which have not been long established by habit, and disturb those that have. Some people become motionless by great surprise, the fits of hiccup and or ague have been often removed by it, and it even affects the movements of the heart, and arteries; but in our sleep, all external stimuli are excluded, and in consequence no surprise can exist.

18. _Why we forget some dreams and not others._

We frequently awake with pleasure from a dream, which has delighted us, without being able to recollect the transactions of it; unless perhaps at a distance of time, some analogous idea may introduce afresh this forgotten train: and in our waking reveries we sometimes in a moment lose the train of thought, but continue to feel the glow of pleasure, or the depression of spirits, it occasioned: whilst at other times we can retrace with ease these histories of our reveries and dreams.

The above explanation of surprise throws light upon this subject. When we are suddenly awaked by any violent stimulus, the surprise totally disunites the trains of our sleeping ideas from these of our waking ones; but if we gradually awake, this does not happen; and we readily unravel the preceding trains of imagination.

19. _Sleep-talkers awake with surprise._

There are various degrees of surprise; the more intent we are upon the train of ideas, which we are employed about, the more violent must be the stimulus that interrupts them, and the greater is the degree of surprise. I have observed dogs, who have slept by the fire, and by their obscure barking and struggling have appeared very intent on their prey, that showed great surprise for a few seconds after their awaking by looking eagerly around them; which they did not do at other times of waking. And an intelligent friend of mine has remarked, that his lady, who frequently speaks much and articulately in her sleep, could never recollect her dreams in the morning, when this happened to her: but that when she did not speak in her sleep, she could always recollect them.

Hence, when our sensations act so strongly in sleep as to influence the larger muscles, as in those, who talk or struggle in their dreams; or in those, who are affected with complete reverie (as described in the next Section), great surprise is produced, when they awake; and these as well as those, who are completely drunk or delirious, totally forget afterwards their imaginations at those times.

20. *Remote causes of sleep.*

As the immediate cause of sleep consists in the suspension of volition, it follows, that whatever diminishes the general quantity of sensorial power, or derives it from the faculty of volition, will constitute a remote cause of sleep; such as fatigue from muscular or mental exertion, which diminishes the general quantity of sensorial power; or an increase of the sensitive motions, as by attending to soft music, which diverts the sensorial power from the faculty of volition; or lastly, by increase of the irritative motions, as by wine, or food; or warmth; which not only by their expenditure of sensorial power diminish the quantity of volition; but also by their producing pleasureable sensations (which occasion other muscular or sensual motions in consequence), doubly decrease the voluntary power, and thus more forcibly produce sleep.

Another method of inducing sleep is delivered in a very ingenious work lately published by Dr. Beddoes. Who, after lamenting that opium frequently occasions restlessness, thinks, "that in most cases it would be better to induce sleep by the abstraction of stimuli, than by exhausting the excitability;" and adds, "upon this principle we could not have a better soporific than an atmosphere with a diminished proportion of oxygen air, and that common air might be admitted after the patient was asleep."

If it should be found to be true, that the excitability of the system depends on the quantity of oxygen absorbed by the lungs in respiration according to the theory of Dr. Beddoes, and of M. Girtanner, this idea of sleeping in an atmosphere with less oxygen in its composition might be of great service in epileptic cases, and in cramp, and even in fits of the asthma, where their periods commence from the increase of irritability during sleep.

Sleep is likewise said to be induced by mechanic pressure on the brain in the cases of spina bifida. Where there has been a defect of one of the vertebræ of the back, a tumour is protruded in consequence; and, whenever this tumour has been compressed by the hand, sleep is said to be induced, because the whole of the brain both within the head and spine becomes compressed by the retrocession of the fluid within the tumour. But by what means a compression of the brain induces sleep has not been explained, but probably by diminishing the secretion of sensorial power, and then the voluntary motions become suspended previously to the irritative ones, as occurs in most dying persons.

Another way of procuring sleep mechanically was related to me by Mr. Brindley, the famous canal engineer, who was brought up to the business of a mill-wright; he told me, that he had more than once seen the experiment of a man extending himself across the large stone of a corn-mill, and that by gradually letting the stone whirl, the man fell asleep, before the stone had gained its full velocity, and he supposed would have died without pain by the continuance or increase of the motion. In this case the centrifugal motion of the head and feet must accumulate the blood in both those extremities of the body, and thus compress the brain.

Lastly, we should mention the application of cold; which, when in a less degree, produces watchfulness by the pain it occasions, and the tremulous convulsions of the subcutaneous muscles; but when it is applied in great degree, is said to produce sleep. To explain this effect it has been said, that as the vessels of the skin and extremities become first torpid by the want of the stimulus of heat, and as thence less blood is circulated through them, as appears from their paleness, a greater quantity of blood poured upon the brain produces sleep by its compression of that organ. But I should rather imagine, that the sensorial power becomes exhausted by the convulsive actions in consequence of the pain of cold, and of the voluntary exercise previously used to prevent it, and that the sleep is only the beginning to die, as the suspension of voluntary power in lingering deaths precedes for many hours the extinction of the irritative motions.